OUR DANCE WITH DEMENTIA

Our Dance With Dementia, A Daughter's Journal © 2015
Kim Kirschenfeld

Printed in the United States of America

Library of Congress Control Number: 2015940491

Paperback ISBN: 978-1-936940-32-5

Design and Printing by Epigraph Publishing Service

Epigraph Books
22 East Market Street, Suite 304
Rhinebeck, NY 12572
www.epigraphps.com

OUR DANCE WITH DEMENTIA

A DAUGHTER'S JOURNAL

KIM KIRSCHENFELD

Epigraph Books
Rhinebeck, NY

CONTENTS

PROLOGUE

This is a book about Paradox—the rich, often humorous, wholly horrifying and confounding paradox that I encountered and engaged in combat with while caring for my mother afflicted with Alzheimer's disease. This book is about the dualities of that disease and about one daughter's process of coping, through awareness and compassion, I hope, but also through humor and satire.

The disease is ugly. It is malevolent, insidious, stealthy and always stalking. In painful slow motion, it poaches and pickpockets the minds of our elders until the cognitive kidnapping is complete and suddenly the parent we knew has become an impostor or at the very least a shuffled version of their former self. In our case, Alzheimer's also freed our mother from the snug constraints of a firmly set mind in a tightly wrapped world of rules and social expectations. The disease's greatest paradox is its cruel fate and the vulnerable beauty that fate can reveal.

This book was initially written as a rather selfish means of expression. My need and my need alone to spill— somewhere—my contradicting emotions of bravado and fear, of duty and denial, of anger and healing, all as tangled and matted as the mixed-up electrons misfiring in my mother's ailing brain. Then, as I "spilled" on paper, her endearing, whacky words amused and enlightened me—the way she combined unrelated words in astonishingly profound ways. The concepts of 'assisted living' and 'memory care' became very real to me. The people involved in her new world of institutionalized living became characters, then stories formed and had to be told.

It is now my attempt to open a dialogue with others who find themselves like me, moving through this Big Mystery invited by cosmic misfortune. I hope in some way to contribute to the universal conversation about our once vibrant, tenacious parents who are now losing sensibilities, who no longer can live at home, or cannot live with us and who perhaps simply live too long...or live differently...or cease to 'live' at all.

Beginning

Maybe it was the day I saw her pluck something from under the kitchen sink—a stiff, forgotten dishrag frayed with dirt and time. After hissing in her Southern sovereign way its urgent need to be thrown away, she nonchalantly spun around on her heels and blew her nose in it. Hard!

I was stunned. *This* from a woman who warned me as a thirsty child in a public place to keep my mouth safely a thumb-length away from the unscoured water fountain spout. A woman, who with righteous indignation, demanded that I scrub my tiny hands every single time after handling a dollar bill because, "you just don't know where it has been."

Or it could have been the afternoon I arrived for our weekly lunch date. My mother answered the front door all ready to go, smiling broadly through pink painted lips and dressed primly in her favorite silk paisley blouse bowed to perfection at the neck. She wore pearls and matching ear bobs that framed her signature 'up-do' anchored well with Aqua Net Extra Hold. She was entirely naked from the waist down.

After I walked her back to the bedroom closet and gently asked if she needed anything else, I noticed that the mirror she used was mounted above her dresser and cut off her reflection exactly at the waist. That explained the half-body ensemble. It took some cajoling, a guessing game of sorts, but she finally looked down and giggled, "Oh dear, my pants."

But it was likely this befuddled response she gave later that day during lunch to my ahhh-isn't-this-nice comment, "It's just you and me, Mama": "*Who is me?*"

My mother has advanced dementia (a super loopy swirl of Alzheimer's and vascular dementia), and the day I realized it matters less. My formerly spunky, downright obstinate, opinionated mother finally succumbed to this sick cluster of symptoms that elusively grows, spawns and breeds unnoticed, denied. Then one day it shamelessly announces itself by a family kitchen sink with the same assertion and supremacy that once described the thoughts and memories it slowly, systematically steals. Without bothering to look back, it leaves those of us around it stranded in its wake, reaching for a safety rope that simply is not there.

Five years ago, a cerebral vascular accident involving my mom, a steep wooden staircase and an unsympathetic marble floor landed her in the hospital and prompted us to consider assisted living. We did. After several years of round-the-clock care in her home of half a century, we moved her to a nearby '5 Star' Memory Care Facility (MC), which seemed like a sound option for a widowed parent showing neurological signs of decline. The young administrator had proudly promoted his new facility as "state of the art" and "built by *resort* developers." I was thinking, yeah, resort developers now in the more profitable business of constructing aesthetically pleasing maximum-security dwellings for old folks with money. Resort developers—as if the notion of a holiday vacation could somehow create the impossible image of Alzheimer's patients hitting eighteen holes of golf and tooling around in golf carts with caddies. Come to think of it, the health aid workers do wear khaki shorts and navy blue golf shirts embroidered with the facility logo that begins with a bulging cursive capital 'A' bobbing across their left breast.

It worked. Or it worked relatively well. I emphasize *relatively* because after the mega-stroke Mama endured prior to admission to The Avery, her physician and well-meaning adult children collectively believed it would be only a few more months before she slipped the surly bonds of Earth and what a nice, immaculate, supportive, convenient facility in which to convalesce…in the meantime.

Now, two years later at eighty-nine and stroke-prone, "her constitution is strong," as one MC nurse at the resort puts it. And I, for one, cannot resolve the guilt long enough to accept that when she does go peacefully to the other side, it will be some random health aid worker in a navy blue golf shirt who finds her, tries to jostle her awake, softly calls her name or who respectfully lowers the eyelids of my mother's moribund body, only to encounter an enduring stubbornness that keeps flipping them open. Her willpower always packed a wallop! My mother never made it easy to be her daughter and this defiance of the odds of death is no exception.

So, as a budding empty nester in her early fifties rumbling around in a deserted, quiet house after a laudable twenty-five-year career of healthy indulgence in the task of mothering, what do I choose to do? The only thing that could impermanently fill that self-imposed emotional void left by the ready exit of three successfully launched young adults; that void left by the proud and underappreciated occupation of Maternal Service. Of course…mother again!

Mimi moved in on Monday.

MOVING

I had acknowledged to Mama for weeks like all the books suggested, that she soon would be leaving her friends at The Avery (with Alzheimer's, every person everyday is a new friend) and her kind caregivers to move in with me. This news, however, failed to elicit the response I had expected. In fact it failed to elicit any response at all. "We-e-ell...," the word stretching itself out and slowly sinking down the memory hole was all I got. Neutral. Indifferent. Unimpressed.

My husband tried to cheer me up at that point. "Oh she will be so happy to have you around...to settle into her new room...to watch seagulls fly over the water from her window...her new hospital bed...shower chair..."

Silence. Some rethinking. Then, "Ok, let's just go."

The movers had finished their work, doing well I might add not to stare curiously at Miss Irene picking wildly at Mr. Bernstein's sweater then screaming in delight. The movers seemed nonplussed when Miss Jean, the Exit Seeker, clutching her big square yellow handbag, tried to body block their way out in order to position herself in an open doorway—her twelfth attempted escape of the day.

Mama's belongings were loaded, her bedroom suite with glorified crown moulding, millwork and twelve foot ceilings now barren, vacated, much like the bankrupt memory of it she left behind. I turned out the light, nudged her walker within reach and with my hand to her elbow, we slowly made our way one last time through the circular garden and into the 'great' room to politely bid our goodbyes.

In the 'great' room (Avery speak for day holding), the movie *Mary Poppins* was warbling from the oversized flat screen mounted above the homey red brick fake fireplace. On the mantle, always seasonally decorated, was a tangle of bright purple, green and gold Mardi Gras beads and boas draping, at times choking, plastic masks smiling eerily beneath empty eyeholes. The scene never seemed to change: two straight rows of eight identical leather Reclina-Rocker La-Z-Boy chairs arm to arm, theatre style, today facing a young Julie Andrews with a black umbrella belting out something about a spoon full of sugar. The Lazies, as we called them, were occupied by a total of six seniors, all overly beaded in purple, green and gold. All were in various stages of industrial sleep: Miss Bettye snoring loudly, Miss Agnes and Miss Margie Flo slumped to their right side in a comfortably warped pile of jumbled anatomy. And I took a deep breath. And I thought, age curves us, one way or another.

I then spotted Mr. Nussman (men in Memory Care kept last names). He was awake, pacing circles around a random chair, but awake. "Mr. Nussman," I say in my louder, Avery voice, "Mimi wants to say goodbye." Under his breath he mumbles, "Where's the damn post office." Without skipping a beat, I reply, "The post office is not in this building as far as I know," and with the dogged optimism of a blind beggar, I try again. "Mr. Nussman, would you like to tell Mimi goodbye?" He ignores me. He ambles toward the muffin tray.

A few feet away, Mama reaches for the arm of an empty Lazy Boy, a reflexive move, and begins to lower herself as always in slow-mo. I catch her and remind her ('mind' actually, there are no 'res' anymore) that we are leaving. She eyes Mr. Nussman. She smiles. Then suddenly, matter-of-factly, she responds to his last comment, "Oh, I've been down cellar too!"

Such are the conversations among Avery mates. And who's to say that this is not some working communication privy only to those elders who have perhaps had enough of timed, earthly linguistic units; elders who simply move on to more complex language, a kind of dateless perpetuity of words. Meanings to the superannuated, they are all just silver threads among the gold. I may be grasping now. I need to go.

An aid worker graciously hugs Mama and perceptively reassures her naive but determined daughter that Mimi's send-off lunch was nothing short of spectacular, a remarkable celebration, and Mimi "enjoyed it so much." I feel better. No, I don't.

Alzheimer's disease makes it okay to leave your home of two whole years without exchanging goodbyes with the people who have bathed you, fed you, dressed you up, held the watercolor brush in your hand at a converted dining room table every Monday morning during arts and crafts hour and signed your initials for you. It's okay to move away from the home you have finally learned your way around without even noticing person, place or thing—or Mardi Gras mask. Just moving on with a prompt of the person beside you.

The rules have changed and for whatever reason I keep on trying, with my mighty, functional mind, to insert the old ones into my mother's life. The old rules that staunchly dictated her etiquette driven pre-Alz life, built on one sturdy-ass foundation of Southern social graces. My mother is now contentedly demented and that has to be good enough for me.

Mimi did not grow up in the South like we did. She grew *into* the South starting about age twenty-two, adopting its ways like a dreamy duckling imprinting the patterns of an old bird dog. She called herself a transplant from *Up*state New York, never just New York. It was necessary in Mimi's healthy mind to stress that two-letter first syllable as if to artificially elevate the whole word; sort of like using 'heirloom' before tomato. But that's the kind of feat that made Mimi the accomplished social athlete she was. Affectation was her sport. Appearance was her silver medal.

Until dementia washed all that away. Until my siblings and I watched things like judgment and pretense slowly dissolve like a melting cube of ice pounded by the force of hot water as it swirls helplessly down an open drain. What was left behind we nurtured. What was left behind was a softer, sweeter, more spontaneous mom.

I bid goodbye on her behalf to the caregivers, as they were the only humans available in a neuro-state other than REM sleep. I turn to press the four-digit security code indelibly etched in my brain. It buzzes loudly, unlocks and releases Mama (and mostly me) forever from state-of-the-art institutional care.

HOME

Barely a quarter mile down the highway toward home, Mama begins her ritual of reading road signs. "Antique Mall, Open Everyday eight to eight." Echoing bad commercial TV, she reads billboards with the manufactured passion of a veteran voice-over actor. "Dirty Carpet? Call Today." Wearing rotund black Chanel sunglasses propped up by the fleck of a nose and swallowing up her frail, narrow face, she continues, "Car Wash with *free* vacuum."

Always on the same side of the road because she is happy looking out only one way, she makes her next surprising announcement: "Pete's UnderCar Care, We Repair," which rolls right into, "Chow Time Grill and Buffet." "Yep" is about all I muster.

Pause. The silence is interrupted by this exciting street sign revelation (and how can her eyesight be so good?): "Magnolia Manor Drive!" Next, as if we have all gone blind, and this time off the side of a passing truck, "Coastal Insulation, call nine. One. Six. Seven. Three…" The truck has sped away.

Depending on the day, I may road sign read with her. It takes me back twenty years to when my kids were buckled up in car seats behind me. Helping Mimi sound out words and explaining that yes, these are signs that businesses use to encourage consumers to buy things they do not need, is a fond maternal memory. But today, impatience rules and I begin to breathe deeply in order to cope with the constant prattle. Until I hear her say, slightly aghast, "Uh oh, uh ohhhhh, oh dear, this NEVER happens." I glance at my husband. He knows. I know. Then quietly, demurely she pleads, "I have to go."

My husband's expression does not change. He does not utter a word. As if on cue, he pulls into Wendy's on our left (incidentally the same Wendy's I used for the same purpose last week). Bowel timing is finely tuned at age eighty-nine.

Without looking, I reach back for Mama's "lady pants" (my ridiculous term, she hardly cares), which are tucked and ready in the pocket behind the passenger seat along with a travel packet of flushable wipes. And we do what we have grown accustomed to doing whenever distance and Mimi are involved. Bathrooms have become venues of togetherness for vast amounts of time and respectful assistance with gastrointestinal functions of eldership.

The enterprise requires me to slow down, to practice patience, to feel humility, to tame a hypersensitive gag reflex, to give back to my mother the years she spent helping me while I was in diapers—my two to her four years and counting but still...

We make it. Adult caregivers have the routine down to a reasonable science: the exact angle to lean a full-grown sitting body for optimal support and access; quick flushes; extra thick wipes; latex gloves if you have them; robotic sequence of clothing removal including shoes and nylon knee-highs one at a time, to make way for the new lady pant; proper disposal of the old; hand washing to the tune of 'Happy Birthday to You.'

Mission complete. As we exit Wendy's, I smile apologetically at the counter employee who barely noticed us handicap-hustling our way in. I am surprised when Mama grabs my forearm, looks up at me from her tiny bent body and whispers loudly in my direction, "Now honey do you have to go? Cause I can help you." And I think, maternal empathy dies hard.

Mimi was an attentive, albeit controlling mother. Parenting for me has been more of an erudite endeavor (one could argue equally contrived) involving far too many books and postgraduate degrees. Sure, there are aspects of my parenting style that reflect my mother's, but I like to think I salvaged only the sound, uninjurious ones and jettisoned the wretched ones that tend to produce defective children. My offspring may of course disagree.

But Mimi was very much a product of her era. She endured just enough nursing school to meet an eligible doctor, jitterbug her way into his heart, marry him, kiss him off to war, and dutifully yield a tribe of five well-spaced, well-behaved reproductions of herself. Because that is just what you did after the second great war, especially in the South where booming babies was all the rage.

Hired help seven days a week was also all the rage in Montgomery, Alabama in the 1950s. And looking back, I owe a huge debt of gratitude to Annie Ruth, whose humming was as deep as a well and wrapped me in a coverlet of calm. To Lula, who proudly nourished us with her fancy peach cobbler and secret-recipe lemon meringue. To Roosevelt, who kept Miss Mimi happy by keeping her azaleas, camellias and crape myrtles watered and pruned. I regret that I never looked them up long after college, that it took me nineteen years to learn their last names. While they were as influential to my upbringing as the second grade teacher who taught me to read, Annie Ruth, Lula and Roosevelt silently blended into my essence the way minerals organically combine to form rock. They each taught me values of hard work, humility, respect and unconditional love without ever trying to; the quintessential teachers who merely model the lesson. To Mimi, they were valued assistance, to me they were tender saviors.

I went to Annie Ruth's house once when I was very young. I remember being intrigued by the sight of her baby daughter sitting upright on a cardboard box to boost her high enough to eat shucked peas at the kitchen table. I was tall enough at my house to reach the dining table without assistance, but for supper that night, I asked Mama for a box to sit on. My silly request was disregarded as an unexplained product of an active imagination.

But nowadays, Mimi would be just fine with a recycled box positioned squarely on a dining room chair. It would be fine for anyone at any age, because now it would simply be a box to boost a baby or satisfy a curiosity or amuse an adult, just another thing that's "there" simply because someone wanted it to be.

After a good twenty minutes inside the WC of American fast food, Mimi and I return to the car. My husband hoists her back in, buckles her up and we resume our journey.

"Brazilian wax, sixty-two dollars, *wow!*" Highway road sign reading begins again. It must be grounding for Mimi in some way, declaring out loud what she immediately sees around her. Emphatically stating the present (to us, the obvious) gives it momentary life, something Mimi can grasp if only for a second. This is her power now, every bit as real as it is fleeting because 'holding' a word or thought has become a major cognitive hurdle. Reading what's out *there*—this she can do. This connects her to an outside world that is otherwise unfamiliar, one that is passing her by at fifty-five miles per hour.

It is the start-and-stop of an oblivious mind. Or it is the steadiness and security of claiming the present, living now, in this moment. And I wonder, sometimes is it wise to know what to forget?

Mimi seems lighter now. It's not as if cognitive awareness has mass of any kind or weight. But in my mother's case, it added poundage, mental trunks and suitcases packed full of hyper-alertness to who was well-born in her opinion and who was not. She had a kind of naturally heightened mnemonic radar attuned to class order and family genus. And she treated you accordingly.

Those are artifacts now, thankfully. The person in Mimi's orbit, whoever that might be, whatever their history, will be the same as the next, as interesting as the next, and all of this without even a name to distinguish them. I will never forget the random ride Mimi shared with me and an old friend of mine. Jade is a transgender, former drag queen living with AIDS and she simply oozes with profound joy and love for everyone she meets. Mimi sat perfectly happy in the back seat giggling with Jade's rapid-fire stories and joining in the chorus of her animated words. Orchestrated 'amens' from an audience of one, it was my mother's unconditional inclusion like never before. Mimi sees everyone now as a friend, an amusing possibility, an ally in her world of unworried whatevers.

Why it took an abhorrent disease I wish upon *no one* to bring my mother back to her essence of love and acceptance, I will never know. She is much lighter now because she no longer carries the burden of hate, the sinking load of antipathy. From her inauspicious state of mind, Mimi is teaching me (in my apparently auspicious one) the health and blessing within the exercise of letting go, of living lightly, unencumbered, so that the beauty all around us has room and space to set firmly inside us.

My mother's wisdom to forget is my lesson to remember.

SEASHORE

It was only a fifteen-minute ride from The Avery to Thirteen Seashore Drive, Mimi's new address. Although she had been there many times, her arrival inquiry was always the same: "How lovely, and who lives here?" Always followed by: "We do, Mama," but today I added, "and now you do too!" My mother looked up at the house from her car window, the kind of wondrous look that comes from a child ogling tall buildings for the first time. Then she asked while still gazing upward, "How lovely, and who lives here?"

This time my husband repeats the proclamation. Mimi turns around in her seat to face me, lowers her forehead and with eyes lasered on my husband whom she has known for exactly forty-seven years, she says furtively from the left corner of her mouth (slightly smudged with Elizabeth Arden dutch-tulip-pink), "Ya gonna invite *him* in?" I nod. We unload.

Inside the front door are Saltillo tile stairs that spiral up steeply, mercilessly from the foyer to the rest of the house. Not thinking ahead, we built our beach house thirteen years ago to maximize views of the water from every room, never considering the safety of an unsteady elder or the possibility of our own decline. Elevated foundation, no elevator, no conceivable space for an elevator, no window coverings, two sets of stairs inside and one outside as the only exits, three floors of hard, very hard, slick travertine, far too many doors to let the outside in, decks abound, aesthetic railing that would fail to protect anyone or anything from falling over. Not childproofed, not elder-proofed, we never needed it to be—until now. So up the ominous steps we go. More like my husband body-lifting my mother hip-to-hip as I part support/part shove her from behind. From that vantage point, I have to smile. Now Mimi is leaning on the man she rebuked thirty years ago as a thoughtless and presumptuous houseguest because without asking he dared to chill a six-pack of beer in her spic and span refrigerator scrupulously organized by food group.

The second floor is the main living space along with her bedroom and its pair of glass French doors that would taunt even a hardcore hermit deckside. From there, slate stairs descending down, an awfully long way down. The French door in her room is tricky to unlock, one safety feature for now. Not the ideal layout for our matriarchal golden-ager, it makes me think about how we structure and organize our homes in direct reflection of our psyches.

My childhood home was a pleasant place most of the time. It was large enough to afford me extended (unnoticed) time and protracted solitude in the inner-sanctum of my pale pink bedroom with its low pile rose colored carpet and wooden sash shuddered windows. I shared the room with three Barbie and Ken families, sometimes four depending on the family constellation I chose that day. They all resided inside a tall white bookshelf laid on its side (Mimi's idea) to make it low enough for me to reach all stories. They lived in tiny square rooms partitioned off by the shelves themselves or improvised walls of cardboard that came back from the dry cleaners in my father's folded shirts. Barbie and family dined and slept on miniature furniture inspired by empty thread spools and overturned paper cups. Soft packing foam sheets became beds and plush carpet samples made perfect pint sized rugs. Their quilts came from old cloth napkins and fabric remnants trimmed in tiny zigzag patterns with a pair of Sears and Roebuck pinking shears.

The families grew sisters and brothers, uncles and aunts as Mattel manufactured their derivatives over time—same face, same body, just different hair, maybe a thinner streak of black eyeliner on the later model, mysterious and redheaded Midge. Even Skipper eventually found friends with the newly marketed Scooter, then Tootie and Todd whose arms could fantastically bend.

My Barbies were my refuge. I got to choose their clothes, their shoes, whether they wore polka dot or plaid, wore high-heels or went barefoot. I chose when to pierce their ears with straight pins or trim their pine straw hair to make bangs or a pageboy. I made all the decisions. It is where I practiced personalities, tried on traits I never dared express outside Barbie-land. It was my interior kingdom of complete control, a place to emulate my mother. I spent hours behind a closed bedroom door. To Mimi, I was conveniently occupied. I played so well by myself, she would brag.

But now it is Mimi who has the sunlit bedroom in someone else's house where she can thrive in a singular imaginary world. The boundaries have blurred, all the people she has known for eighty-nine years, memories she has stored in the drawer of her mind enter and exit at will. She merely follows their lead.

Imagination and reality stir together for Mimi now and their concoction is the one-dimensional moment her supple life has become. She lives openly now in ways she could not have imagined or appreciated before. There is no need for avoidance now, no need to escape, no fear of anything 'other,' no longer is there an 'us' and 'them.' Tenderly faded borders of thought have liberated Mimi and permitted her to unlock critique of herself and those around her. Unafraid, she welcomes in a benevolent outside world.

"Welcome Home Miz Mimi," Bell rejoices from another room. Nineteen years before, Pinkie Bell Putnam winged her way into our lives like a wide girthed, black fairy godmother belching out Bible verses and gospel hymns. She charged through the back kitchen door of our first home in town the day after my husband and I moved there with three small children and a truckload of belongings. In a gust of goodwill and almighty dominion, Bell barged on in and without looking, nailed the wall peg with her giant pocketbook and announced her name and vocation as our new nursemaid. She came with the house so to speak.

The previous owner had employed her for years, and personally, I was relieved and grateful to have unsolicited help with a seven-year-old, a three-year-old and a newborn. Bell quickly became family (and deep sleeping babysitter I was later told by my seven-year-old). She got to know Mimi during the lucid years, so it was only natural that Bell would help manage my mother's essential needs through the less lucid ones.

Bell double-dared her own seventy-eight big, beautiful years to "take holda MY brain!" and it worked. She was spry, plucky and downright bossy in advanced age. Bathing in her glory, Bell allegiantly ruled Thirteen Seashore, and to her, my mother was just one more divine soul sent to her in need of service—a holy gift the Good Lord bestowed onto Pinkie Bell Putnam for free.

We had barely cleared the last perilous stone step when Bell elbowed my husband out of her way and practically airlifted my frail, confused one hundred-pound mother to her favorite Stickley rocking chair by the window overlooking the water. "There you be Miz Mimi, Bell gone git ya Hershey Bar." She knew my mother well. On the way to her chocolate stash, thumping that barrel chest of hers, Bell sang to the air as if praising with her Tenth Street True Gladness Choir, "Religion's right here in your heart, Miz Mimi, ain't jest on your knees."

Genuine Glorification of the Holy Ghost meets Happy Go Lucky Lunacy. This just might work.

MORNINGS

Bell arrives when Bell arrives, but always early enough. This morning while pecking away on my laptop keyboard, I hear the front door open, then slam. Heavy footsteps and a low hum of gospel song. It feels like church just walked through my front door—a sanctified blessing by osmosis.

Plates begin to collide with the cupboard shelf, then the clamor of cookware on the stone counter. More humming, with emphasis this time. The whir of blending batter, then that dense, creamy waft of Bell's yellow butter pound cake trailing up from the warm kitchen oven below. Pound cake iced with hot melting confectionery sugar dribbling to transparency along its rim—one more culinary virtue that Bell and Mimi share. It is fructose liquefaction, sweet nectar of the Southern cake baking gods!

My mother used to bake for love. Because words were not as easy, triple chocolate brownies had to suffice. Homemade cookies and fanatically decorated cupcakes became her carefully measured expressions of loving us. Desserts with every meal. So I have to believe that this familiar ambrosia of baking aromas floating through the house somehow, on some cell level, calms Mama's whirl of neuro-commotion.

And it does. I hear Bell's deep melodic harmony of words, "Miz Mimi, c'mone and sit with your shugga donut." I walk down to greet them both and see Mimi first. Buttoned up in a wool coat as if she's about to brave an indoor blizzard, Mimi is barefoot and appears puzzled. I watch. Standing still in the middle of the room with her eyes closed, she inhales audibly, snorts really, then shakes her head in exasperation. "I declare, I left my oven on again. Quick, my lemon supreme!"

Oh the sweet, unforgettable scent of a cake once made. That intimate amalgamation of white bleached flour, two hearty cups of real butter and processed sugar that, for a moment, reacquainted my mother's senses and her brain. And maybe gently awakened a memory or two. Bell beats her to the hot oven but lets her peek inside. "Thaz right Miz Mimi, es almost done." Mimi relaxes; she is pleased.

When home on breaks from college thirty years ago, my sister and I would sarcastically refer to the room where cooking is done as "her kitchen." Mimi ran a tight ship, an organized food facility. Meals were served at designated hours, we learned early on that snacking and grazing were strictly prohibited.

"The kitchen is closed!" she would screech from a distant room. "She has bat hearing," my older sister would whisper as she slammed the refrigerator door and dashed away from the front line of Mimi's wrath. Those frosty words from my mother made me freeze in place, shamefully busted with Waterford crystal cake dome in hand. The seductive assortment of pastel baby petit fours inside was not to be eaten at leisure. They were Mimi-earmarked for a certain meal, or guest. Latent eating disorders be damned!

Meal planning in Mimi's house was a calculated operation, a fall-in at The Citadel. Basic training regs: one hand in the lap while dining, elbows hidden below the table at all times, chewing had to be slow, preferably with lips sealed, no Army-eating and under no circumstances could one 'talk with their hands.' In fact, talking at all about controversial topics while dining like, say, current events, world state of affairs, real things happening to real people, would be called out and accused—evidence of one's failure to prove they had what it took to be part of Mimi's table platoon.

So naturally, today in my family kitchen, Mama sits at a table formally set for one. Perched upright and patient, a half eaten Little Debbie powdered donut on a bone china plate before her, she painstakingly dabs each corner of her mouth with a stiff white linen napkin, knowingly starched by Bell. She is dressed for the Arctic region in winter, yet Mimi still has table manners that would make Emily Post proud.

"Good morning, Mama," is followed by her shocked and wide-eyed response to me, "What in the world are YOU doing here?" "I live here," is my reply. Unconvinced, my mother puts down her donut, refolds the linen in her lap and shoots out, "Now stop that!" Pause. "But you can use the place anytime." She returns to her donut. "OK, thanks," is all I can say. We move on.

I give her a kiss on the cheek and remind her that my brother, her beloved only son, is coming to visit later today. Donut down again, "Well…I'll have to wait for Jack you know." My father (Jack) died eight years ago but apparently checks in with my mother on a routine basis. I assure her that will be fine and that her son won't mind a bit waiting for her.

"Well...I may not be back by then," she warns, looks away and finishes that last little crumb of artificial nougat.

So I bring my mother a juicy, seasonal Ruby Red grapefruit, quartered just like mine. And in silence we spoon our citrus and sip our coffee. Nothing in particular to say, nothing in particular to solve and nothing in particular for Mimi to criticize, just slowly sharing breakfast at our round family table, side by side.

It's easy. Mimi looks happy. I smile.

OUTBREAK

"She's on the warpath!" This was code my sister used when we were kids to warn me about Mimi's temperament on any given day. It also meant that my sister was on her way out the door in her 1972 tripped out GTO with its vinyl landau roof and newfangled 8-track tape player inside.

For me, it meant rapid retreat to my upstairs bedroom. Behind a closed door, I might grab a ready stenographer pad, blank with possibility, and become Della Street, the glamorous gal Friday I watched on Perry Mason reruns. She was smart and efficient with her dark silhouette of tailored suits and pencil skirts. She was a place I could go, a more age-appropriate step above Barbie-land, to pretend away the thundering tirade brewing a floor below.

Mimi could be wicked. I heard my father politely describe it as irritability or going against the grain. "Relaaaax," he would advise her, with futility. Whatever it was, in the early 1970s, no one was in a hurry to diagnose it and everyone close to me was dashing to avoid it. Each of us learned early to take shelter in strategy. Holing up with my dolls and character roles in the safe harbor of imagination was mine. My sister made mileage down the road of denial with a hyper-social personality and too many afterschool commitments.

My brother found solace with stringed instruments and my oldest sisters were away at college, safely out of the line of fire. When I heard music of Rachmaninoff blasting from behind the bi-fold door of my father's study, I knew he was nestled inside with a book and tobacco pipe.

In the midst of any madcap moment, Mimi said things she had to later regret. Once when I left an unmade bed behind before her guests arrived on Sewing Circle day, Mimi pierced me with this: "You couldn't do that for *me*? I suffered labor pains for *you*!" It worked. At age eleven, I took full responsibility for my own procreation and felt badly for being born. I remember sleeping with a fluffy pillow not under but over my head in case a late night rant at high pitch had to be hushed. This was long, long before earbuds and iDistractions.

I never fully understood what stoked the red-hot embers of my mother's wire coat hanger rage. It spewed without warning, dousing mostly my dad. But even when Rachmaninoff was loud, Mimi's verbal weaponry still launched like a long-range unguided missile, target unknown.

Now, Mimi is no more capable of hurling a hateful word as she is of slalom skiing behind a speedboat. I believe the pliable Mimi before me is the essential one. The one who willingly cupped all her coins in my five-year-old hand so I could proudly present them to a paraplegic beggar we passed on a street one Sunday afternoon in 1963. This Mimi is the one who emerged and quietly asked me if I would mind sharing a few of my get-well gifts with a fellow Children's Hospital patient she surmised was indigent and without family support.

These moments of humanity unveiled by my mother are the memories that cling and smooth the chipped edges of my childhood. While most daughters of dementia feel they lose a parent to the ravages of disease, I paradoxically found mine. And I recognize her now from the compassionate acts I vividly recall that number less but mean so much more than the wounding ones I would rather forget.

It is possible that Mimi never realized that she deserved to be happy, that she was capable of letting light in to eclipse all the shadows. Her private villains that seemed to lacerate her soul curbed her into a darkness where she tended to resist exactly what she needed most—uncut human connection.

Somewhere along the way, Mimi stumbled from the weight of her anger, hobbled from the heft of her pain. And it is not easy to stand up again. But now, bent with age and degeneration, Mimi is standing. She has found footing in the oddest of ways. As this dreaded disease quarantined my mother's mind, it also locked out the turbulence. And as her healthy mind waned like a slowly decomposing carcass, so too did her unwanted anger. I believe when a mind is whittled down this far to its seminal nature, there simply is no lie left to carry. So, with an openheartedness I know was always deep within, she has now taught me to let go and love.

WORDS

Today my mother made up another new word. Sparch. While sitting peacefully together in the warm morning sunshine—me reading our local newspaper, Mimi dozing on and off cocooned tightly at her request in a creamy beige fleece blanket—she blurted out, "Sparch."

"What's that?" I peer over my 2.0 readers propped on the end of my nose. Silence. Mimi silence, her eyes wandering across the deep blue vista of the Santa Rosa Sound drifting below us. Calm water gleaming in sunlight like iridescent scales on the skin of a fish. I can tell she is trying to find her new word again. "What is Sparch, Mama?" A sigh. Then in a sudden burst of clarity, "Well, it means we are different than we were before."

I stop reading. I put down the paper and join her gaze, watching water. And we absolutely are, aren't we?

In the nakedness of that moment, I think about my mother's daisy chain of words. Years ago when the brain blundering began, she said to me, "I get something in my mind, then I don't remember it. I can't remember if I remember it or not." And I think it must be a bit like barely controlled falling. First, a thought occurs. It is real. Then it begins to slide off some wet, glossy edge of slippery gray matter into a cool, shallow puddle of sounds…somewhere. Maybe then, that thought splashes around, having fun for a nano-second with other easygoing sounds that have also detoured south. Then, one or two or even three words fall out of the mouth miraculously still attached to those other sounds like braided strays of meanings. These might form some liquidy blend of a new watery word. All in a matter of cerebral seconds. Wow.

Or maybe there is intelligible meaning that I, in my less evolved state of wisdom, simply fail to decipher. This could be our one opportunity as dementia daughters to dive deeply, head first, with our mothers into our cell co-psyches, into the scary helixes of our shared DNA, to grapple *together* amid our common coils and meet halfway to finally begin to understand the other.

If she could have said it at that moment, I would have heard, "I do not know your name but I know I love you."

Love and language. Sparch. I close my eyes like Mimi and decide to nap hard.

Bundling

Mimi likes to bundle things. Not like the cable and internet bill, but like a mismatched pair of nylon knee-highs stuffed with silver wrapped chocolate kisses and knotted tightly at the top. Repurposed knee-highs might be bunched with a five by seven framed photograph of herself, three stray clip-on earrings and a blue ballpoint pen, all snugly wrapped together inside a small-medium undergarment for adults. In order to keep her good gaggle intact, Mimi binds it like a bale of hay with red curling ribbon she has stashed in the back of her lingerie drawer.

This bundle du jour is smaller than the one she made yesterday. For that one, she used her wool blended winter coat as the vessel for a bath towel, two washcloths, a toothbrush and a book about wolves. When I saw this swollen lump of apparel, I thought of a headless Quasimoto wearing my mother's coat, bent over into a ball. Mimi's saddlebag of today's gear is ready for departure, making her souped up four wheel Rollator walker the getaway freight car.

She has stacked each tight bundle atop the double padded seat of her walker and lets lighter cargo dangle from both airbrake handles. At the bottom is her handy tote basket brimming with household booty from the linen closet. It is an activity that Mimi engages in when she has too much time on her hands. "I gotta go!" is what I hear as I wiggle through the sliver of her open bedroom door now barricaded by her handicapable mode of transport. The walker sits, ready to roll, always right by her door, often next to two brass bedside lamps, shades and bulbs carefully removed, with their gold plastic cords neatly wrapped in rows around their bases. Mimi gently tucks in the outlet prongs of each lamp to prevent unraveling or injury.

Mimi can evacuate a drawer in mere minutes, as long as something remotely resembling a container is nearby. She is resourceful. Socks can be crammed with sunglasses, a comb and a bookmark. Single latex gloves yanked from the box in the bathroom serve as casing for a tube of toothpaste, her Bible, and Oil of Olay moisturizer.

A stack of framed family photographs sits directly on the floor near the getaway walker, tied up with two silk scarves. Her bedroom wall is now barren, with gold picture hangers exposed where the photographs hung earlier today. And yesterday. This has become Mimi's routine since she moved in. Apparently she is preparing to go—somewhere. "I'm almost ready, sweetheart," she advises as I stand in the middle of her room, again thinking how long it will take to put everything back. Mimi's bundles require great care to undo, as the undoer never knows what breakable treasure lies inside and will crash to the floor.

Imagining her answer, I ask the question anyway. "Where are you going today?" And like Dorothy at the entrance to Oz, she cheerfully replies, "Goin' home, Jack will be here any minute." Having long ago surrendered to the futility of anything close to a reality check, I simply ask where home might be. Mimi laughs out loud while frantically wiping out the last empty drawer with the sleeve of her cashmere sweater. "Now don't be silly," she says, and referring to her heavily laden walker she laments, "I gotta hurry up and push my pusher because it is hard to find a place to park."

Going with the flow, I respond, "Traffic is bad this time of day so we could just unpack and sit here for a bit." Oblivious to my suggestion, Mimi picks up the framed photo on top of floor stack number five. It slides out easily from the silk scarf binding. Relieved by her distraction I comment, "That's a picture from my wedding, do you remember it?" Mimi studies the photograph, brushes her hand across its surface and sits down. "Oh, I see you now, and who are the other kids getting married with you?" The bridesmaids and groomsmen do look blissfully wed as well. Confusing.

With nothing more to say on the matter, I smile and notice how the late afternoon sun from Mimi's window illuminates the tiny floating particles of dust in the air we share; particles stirred by the lively buzz of Mimi's need to feel busy, her need to be anything other than idle, her need to feel secure and to find a place that feels like home.

As her daughter I can certainly provide safe shelter, healthy food, compassionate care and pleasant company, but what I cannot give back to her is Boxwood Drive, her home of fifty years and what her life used to be, a home and a life she built with the strength of an ox and the dedication of a monk. What mattered to Mimi—her showplace residence, her crowded social calendar, her travels with Jack, volunteer work at her church—are the things that gave her meaning, things that in my youth I mostly ignored but assumed would define her forever. Like many women of Mimi's generation, work revolved around the state of her home, the wellbeing of her family, the extent of her social agenda. Those former measures of Mimi's worth, so important at the time, have become bits of powdery debris to her, like the specks of dust that free float around her room in the shadow of a setting sun.

Mimi yawns and says she is tired. I help her out of her shoes and overcoat and sweater and scarf and jewels, and suggest a nice afternoon nap. She acquiesces. I lie down beside her and inhale a faint, familiar hint of Jean Patou Joy. With eyes closed, she hits her final hum with a drowsy question, "How do I know if this dream is mine?" "I just don't know, Mama." I listen to the silence until my mother falls asleep. Then I carefully rise and begin to unpack, replace and restore so that when she awakens, her room, her sphere of the moment, might, this time, feel like home.

NATHANIEL

It is interesting how just an otherwise ordinary day that rolls around routinely every year becomes a lifelong marker of time when some horrific event falls within its twenty-four hours. Friday, April 13, 2012. A brilliant, extraordinary, remarkable twenty-six-year-old close friend of my daughter's died suddenly of cardiac arrest.

Nathaniel was my daughter's rock throughout law school. She was his reliable confidante and welcome distraction from the impossible challenges associated with a congenital heart condition. He was to graduate from law school forty-two days after his death.

This was a young man who, wise beyond his years, learned early to cope with risk and pain and the impermanence of life. His limitation did not define him, it propelled him to achieve unparalleled academic success and it fostered iconic courage rarely seen in adults twice his age.

In a letter to me, he wrote about empathy—about its ability to transcend pain, the privilege it allowed a person to understand a situation they had never experienced before. This, he wrote, was his best evidence that pain is not the story of a person's life—things like compassion and empathy are.

My daughter and I had not felt this abysmal depth of despair before April 13th. Healing will be timeless and as unpredictable as Nathaniel's heart. Acceptance, at least for me, may never come. Every day, I now fight the urge to yell at a perfectly innocent, random middle-aged guy on the street, "Why, Sir, do you get to live?" Or for that matter, why do I? My husband tells me that this is the anger stage of grief recovery. *Stage*—that which passes with time. I am not sure that there is a stage to this brand of pain.

Sadness this size, anger this thorough obliterates any well-intended notion of passage of time. The contemptible robbery of a strong, brave, wholly aware young man full of promise who barely eked out two decades of life, leaving behind a world of beloveds just weeks before owning his well deserved law degree, is a merciless, monstrous proposition.

Then there is Mimi—a nonagenarian, chair-bound and incontinent, unable to differentiate her own five grown children from the girl scouts selling Snickerdoodles at her front door. A woman who led a healthy and whole, charmed life spanning nine decades. A woman who is now lost and widowed from the love of her life and whose body refuses to follow the fully human, natural mortification of the mind and who, by the way, vociferously expressed her wishes to more than one of us that she never wanted "to be taken care of" or to live past her ability to contribute and produce and to love back her family.

Another paradox: Some would argue that Mimi's life is a life lived too long but *all* would argue that Nathaniel's was lived too briefly. This disobedience of death, this lawlessness of life simply defies reason. It is blatantly unfair.

Ironically, Mimi, in her healthier years, would wholeheartedly agree. "I never want to be a burden" was a seven word phrase she often hurled in martyr mode. But when she said it, I found it far too easy to dismiss. Because until the mental and physical limitations appear in a parent, imagining what it takes to accommodate them is beyond comprehension. Few options exist besides moving them into a structured environment or hiring care at home if financial means allow it.

Maybe losing our mental faculties is both burden and a gift. Two situations we all want to avoid but fear we are standing in line for, waiting our random turn, at any time we can become caregiver or patient, the gift-giver or gift-receiver. And that last part, for me, involves interchangeable parts. Whether we are providing care or accepting care, we become partners in a dance that turns into a ritual. With no formal training, no practice or rehearsal, we shuffle around together as a pair of sightless sidekicks in some bizarre ensemble of steps that neither of us has ever seen performed.

We are rudely invited to this shindig of sorts and mutually reluctant to attend. But we do. We show up. My mother and I have learned to switch leads now and then in order to adapt to each other's instinctive rhythms. We negotiate new steps and learn this mysterious, haunting routine as we go.

Mourning

Still gripped by the great vise of grief and hiding out like a coward from Happy Humanity, I decide to beseech the wisdom of Mimi.

This morning I find her bundled up by Bell in her favorite knit sweater(s) and swaddled tightly in not one, but two, soft fleece throws. It is sunny, humid and eighty degrees but Mimi's world is cold. She is smiling, looking peaceful, indifferent to the heat and not the least bit sweaty napping in a rocker on the back deck. I quietly sit down in a matching rocker and absentmindedly (runs in the family) synchronize my rocking motion to hers.

She opens her eyes, still smiling. Then, with Mimi's special brand of irrefutable moral certainty, she leans forward and declares quite directly to the atmosphere and me, "Why look at the...uh...those whachamacallits!" "Oh," I interject, "you mean the white blooms on the magnolia tree, you always love magnolias." Apparently perturbed by my false presumption, she suddenly cuts me off. "NO-O-O, you're not looking! Those tops, round and all stirred." "OK," I agree and mention that I see them *now*, to which she replies, "And boy, they are loaded." We rock some more.

I may be hiding out from expressing grief appropriately. I know I am spreading around dark depressive thought, but I have to admit, free-associating conflicted feelings coated in pain to someone physically there but decidedly not has its benefits. I know that using words to describe my despair may help lift its weight and temper its power. So I go for it.

"Mama, Nicolet's close friend died suddenly two weeks ago and I am struggling to accept it. I keep wanting to undo his death. I am angry and insufferable to be around." I swallow the gargantuan lump in the back of my throat. Expressing heartfelt emotion to Mimi never seemed to be an option for me. I generally assumed the more negative the emotion, the more likely it would be ignored. Mimi hears me. She sighs, as if she is contemplating my situation. Could this be the sign of empathy I need? I notice that I am holding my breath. This is foreign terrain for us. "Who, Coco?" (Nicolet's nickname—a spark of recognition!) She continues her thought, "We-e-ell, I'm not anywhere either."

Intrigued, I push on. "Nathaniel was a generous, loving, insightful young man so full of light and laughter, and so smart. Mama, you would have approved." Mimi keeps rocking, staring straight ahead. In the bright sunlight, I notice the fine art of an elder's lined face, creases and rows bending and winding like a tributary of goodness wrapping its way around the source. Each line is like a stream, a tracing of time.

Mimi takes her time and finally replies. "Seems to me he had some pretty good lunches, but this is alright too." He did have those. And eventually, it may be.

Then, without looking, as if sensing the presence of something heavy and out of place, Mimi reaches into her left sweater pocket and pulls out two perfectly smashed, bright yellow Splenda packets obviously snatched from a restaurant where we dined weeks ago. She studies them, turns them over and over, each one receiving her undivided attention. Unimpressed, she slides them back into the other sweater pocket and cranes her neck a bit toward our neighbor's boat lift across the way. Nodding in its direction, Mimi says with a determined tone, "Is that a schoolhouse next door? I have been looking for the flag."

I think for a second. A tragic premature death. The loss of a friend we loved. Unfair fate and who gets to live. I guess I have been looking for something too.

Before nodding off once more, my mother tosses me one more pearl: "I have in my mind it's a Sun afternoon." And I think about how much I love the sun, how it rises every single day with or without us, vital and new and life-giving, a mortal coil of light that invites us in, if we are lucky enough to be around.

Minutes pass—the calm, peace filled ones—and in a surprising way, the quiet alone fills up my hollow heart space of sadness. It is in moments like these that I realize something: Mimi, in her madness, can take me to a place where time is slow and joy is easy enough to find in simple things like watching water or feeling sunshine or looking for flags.

Life ends, unlike mourning, which lives.

FLOWERS

Flowers and Mimi share a common language. To her, they speak of refinement, arrangement, ornamental symmetry and always a delicate photogenic result. But it was also the process of cultivating them that brought her peace.

Mimi always seemed happiest with her bare hands in the dirt. Digging, watering, snipping and planting were all parts of her spiritual work. I remember her on sunny days wearing white peddle pushers, as she called them, a starched, untucked, white cotton shirt with sleeves carefully, evenly rolled, matching visor tipped down, her body bent to the earth. By touching living plants, placing seeds in blooming beds, she found a safe way to nurture life with no risk of rejection. Plants do not talk back, do not resist what they are offered, plants are "handled" and Mimi could do that quite well. When we grow things our hearts fill with hope. Maybe that is why she loved to weed. The inarticulate fury of yanking away decay and debris may have somehow helped to detangle the mystifying roots quite possibly choking her heart.

Mimi was never comfortable sharing with us the details of her childhood. What she did describe, when we asked, was idyllic. What she left out was significant. So I got to fill in the gaps with my imagination, guided by hers. One way she filled in the gaps was by working in her meticulously groomed gardens. A panoply of bright pink azaleas that bloomed in grandeur abundance each spring, neat linear rows of wispy crape myrtle trees, mounds of lacey blue hydrangeas, all painstakingly placed along carefully laid red brick walking paths that wound and circled proficient pine and hardy heritage oak trees—all leading to the stark white, rarely used garden gazebo at the center of her pleasance. Mimi spent more time in her garden than she did with us. And I now understand why. There in her secluded slice of nature, Mimi found quiet and a place to sequester her fundamental spirit of goodness. In that approving space, she touched something elemental and absolute about herself. It was real. She felt intact and protected from anyone out there who might otherwise judge or evaluate her imagined shortcomings.

I am grateful that I am now getting to know this Mimi-In-Her-Garden, the substance of Mimi that I regretfully missed for fifty years. And I consider this the greatest paradox of terminal illness: the uncovered core of a person it reveals, the delinquent *and* gracious invitation to come in. It took Alzheimer's disease to grant Mimi the freedom from a shadow of 'shoulds.' It allowed us to become acquainted as friends at eighty-nine and fifty-three.

In gratitude and in honor of her liaison with all things floral, I like to fill her room with a vase of fresh flowers every week. I am careful to change the water she once would have scoffed at as foul and murky. Sometimes she notices the flowers, often she forgets them and notices them again. Depending on the particular flower, it may bloom, wilt or shed. All phases of that flower's life fascinate my mother now; all are equally splendid in her eyes. There is no need to remove dead petals or dropped leaves anymore. Now Mimi sees through one moment in time. She no longer resists what she cannot control. She sees that with change, with life cycles ending, something new, something lovely can form.

So today, I decided to plant for Mimi and to plant for Nathaniel. I chose a shady corner of our front yard. Mimi sat closely by in a lawn chair while I dug into the dirt and felt the cool earth as she once did. I pressed and settled in a small key lime tree with many green sprouts to be. Mimi held the hose while we soaked roots. She commented on smiling clouds and asked if I wanted a card table for Christmas this year because "the kids are at just the right age." I mentioned that my youngest was in college and away from home and reminded her of Tessa's recent visit and the day they spent together. She furrowed her brow and asked, "Oh? And where was I?"

Mimi continued to hold the garden hose and as her thoughts drifted, so did the nozzle of the hose. She proceeded to spray from her sitting position, every plant and tree and object within striking distance. That included me. Well watered and hysterically laughing, I realized how easily Mimi now takes my heart out to play.

Chuckling along with me but not sure exactly why, Mimi asks me if there is anything she is supposed to be doing. I assure her that she is exactly where she is supposed to be, to which she follows up, "Now I didn't go ahead and get more places, did I?" In earlier days, Mimi had an expensive knack for spotting and buying promising real estate, usually in the form of houses and condominiums. Mimi called them her "places." She decorated and redecorated them as home fashions changed. To Mimi, place meant status, place meant escape, place meant anywhere but where she was. Looking back, she was always on the go, packing and unpacking, traveling and returning. Movement, not stability, was her game, and perhaps it caused enough of a distraction from whatever it was she felt she needed to leave behind.

At the tiny tree's base, I place a large pink conch shell I found at the bottom of the sea. A tree in tribute to not one, but two friends—one young, one old.

And *that* fills my heart with hope.

MOTHERHOOD

Having my grown kids home for vacation, individually or in tandem, is sheer gift. They bring life and laughter and youthful dimension into our house. The youngest, Tessa, home from college in New York, is rummaging through the refrigerator in search of gluten-free breakfast options when Mimi emerges from her bedroom. She is dressed in her Burberry overcoat, tightly buttoned to the top, belted to perfection, her silk "nightie" (her term) underneath, no shoes. She has a distressed look on her face.

"Good morning, Mimi," Tessa says cheerfully and greets her with two open arms and a smile. "What are you doing here?" my mother replies with a direct stare and for a brief moment (aside from the outfit) seems to be engaging in lucid conversation. "I came to visit you, Mimi. I live in New York, close to where you grew up!"

Pause. I look Mimi's way for the next unpredictable move. She seems to relax, perhaps responding to some inkling of familial connection cast lovingly by her favorite grandchild. Her expression softens and in perfect Southern dialect, she says, "Well, I have been here for *over* an hour, honey, trying to get all this stuff ready to go!" "You have?" Tessa replies with ready compassion. Then...Tessa does the unthinkable, says something to me that is inconceivable, outlandish, unspeakable, unforgivable: "Hey Mom."

Mimi stops dead in her tracks. She glances at Tessa and *glares* at me as if I had just ripped the last Little Debbie sugar donut from her hands. My body freezes, an impulsive response born out of fifty years of my mother's trademark hubris defined by that *glare*! As a child, I went into tachycardia when I saw that glare. Mimi takes her time. I feel a cruel comment brewing. I look up wearing childhood shame and she finally strikes: "W-H-Y are YOU everyone's *mother*?"

Phew, so that was it. Another Mimi-ism, but with the added flavor of dementia. But you know, it just does not sting like it used to. Wordless once again, I slightly smile as I notice the futility of my mother's malice these days, the malice she smoked and cured with the salt of her words and saved for anyone or anything that dared to challenge her perception of what should be. But her loaded comment seems insignificant now leaking out from narrow, quivering lips and framed by ivory folds of paper thin skin. Despite the stubborn demise of my mother's handy condemnations—those remaining morsels of malevolent critique of the world that just won't wither away—I notice that the old intimidation is gone. I can see those comments for what they always were, protective weapons against fear—Mimi's fear. Mimi, the late, great adjudicator of all things worthy and well bred. Dementia has a lovely way of dissolving unwanted things like insolence and condescension much like a deluge of rainwater that washes away scattered litter strewn about carelessly and collected haphazardly by a muddy curb.

I help my mother to her favorite rocking chair. Tessa brings her a glass of freshly squeezed orange juice and without asking, proceeds to prepare virtually the same breakfast her grandmother always made for her—two scrambled eggs and one slice of lightly buttered toast.

Tessa's reference to me as "mom" clearly incensed my mother. As if my role as mother-at-large organically evoked some deep, personal feeling that somewhere in the recesses of her fading memory, she recalls *and* she knows she owns and misses. Motherhood—the intensive labor, immeasurable joy, infinite love, occasional disappointment, the heart attachment and the multitude of sacrifices made in its pursuit. Mimi and I share that in common.

Durability of Motherhood. Immortality of Motherhood.

But alas, with Alzheimer's if one encounters an insult, a direct hit, one needs only wait a moment or two. The sensorial tide will quickly change.

MOONS

Mimi's days unroll loosely like the pleasantly wrapped linen serviettes Bell painstakingly irons and over-starches for Mimi's midday meal, the ones Mimi jiggles and shakes, spilling out polished silver flatware onto the mahogany table with a clunk.

Her days are about the same. And they aren't. In Mimi's world, Sundays could be Tuesdays. Fridays, Mondays. She is steeped in the moment she is in, stalled in time. Moment to moment is all Mimi knows now. And I think of another paradox: Dementia is vulnerable beauty; dementia is alarming disturbance—disturbance that clunks down with a thud when we least expect it. It is the sudden screech of a foghorn let go inside a shrine.

There is a Zen koan, a parable, called 'No Moon No Water.' It is about an aging nun, Chiyano, toting river water one night in an old wooden bucket. She looks down into her bucket and notices how the top of her water catches the moon's beautiful reflection. When her weary bucket breaks through from the weight of its contents, the water inside along with the moon disappears onto the ground beneath her feet. It is then that Chiyano realizes her life is like that moon, just an image of something else.

It is a metaphor of course, but if this potency of emptiness, this spiritual state of absence somehow, in some way unites us with Nirvana, then Mimi has quite possibly achieved a near Zen level of enlightenment.

Yesterday, I found her in her bedroom curiously lodged and stuck between a window and her walker. I easily helped her out then asked what she needed. She chuckled in her 'I'm totally fine' way and replied, "W-e-e-l-l, I need to find that broom to sweep up the dingle dangle from the trees outside." I noted that the outside trees were pretty far away. She appeared puzzled because she saw trees with "dingle dangle," and in that single moment, all she knew was that she needed to sweep. Period. I offered to take her outside to get closer to the trees so we could check the dingle dangle and she was satisfied. "Oh that would be nice," was her reply. As we walked, I thought about my own perceptions as mere reflections of something else. Perhaps we all define our realities like Mimi does, and any one is as authentic, as justified, as another.

Walking for Mimi is labored these days; slow, not too steady, but determined. We sit. We look for dingle dangle in trees. Then, without warning, her energy may drastically change. Like today, Mimi becomes agitated for no reason I can find. Nothing I say helps, everything I do annoys. And there it is: a piercing sliver of the inexplicable anger I grew up with and know so well. Today, was it a sudden lucid thought that provoked her anger? Was it her recollection of my plethora of limitations in her mind? Was it simply a quick ride on her cerebral tilt-a-whirl? Or just the darn broom she could never find?

And then it is gone, as quickly as it came. So on these days when I feel helpless, inept at caregiving, depleted by my mother's riveting decrepitude, I try to remember (quite the challenge at the moment, after all I am the product of my genes) that Mimi's thinking is real, but disguised--terra incognita. And when it tends to shift for no reason or vaporize entirely into the ether, she may just be operating at a different mental altitude—perhaps on a plane to Nirvana just like Chiyano, the night sky-toting nun. Just like the moon in a bucket of water.

WAVES

Mimi died in her sleep. Peacefully deep in a colorful, floral dream I hope, and smiling with my dad by her side. Maybe they were swimming in the warm waters of the Gulf of Mexico they loved. Maybe they weren't.

The paradox of my mother's condition reminds me of the paradox of our ocean—horrifying and tender at the same time, capable of both devastating destruction and resurging genesis, threatening and healing all in the same breath. Quite like her final gasp of air.

Those waves we know so well. Those waves mended my parents, my siblings and me together for so many years before we all grew up and navigated our lives away from the source. Those are the same waves my adult children grew up with and still surf and ride when they are home for a visit. It is the same gentle Gulf current that flows through their soul and binds them together and with elders before them.

Those are the waves that crest and crash in syncope, that mark the inevitable rise and fall of life—Mimi's life. And which years were her rise? Which years were her fall? Or does it even matter? It is the coincidence of confusion and clarity that her condition unnaturally combined that put motion to the music of her mind.

Clarity may have led the tarantella. Confusion may have followed. But I have to wonder if those two partners in sync periodically switched positions to provoke and inspire those of us around her, inspired us to feel, to wonder and to love, as they performed and we followed in step, in full dress and decorum for that last, long promenade across the floor.

Either way, I was clearly the beneficiary. Wide-eyed and captive on the first row, engaged and awestruck, sometimes bellowing 'bravos,' other times bewildered into silence by the impossible choreography set to the tunes of Mimi's elusive imagination. Pain and struggle command our full attention. They teach. They strengthen. They also hurt. Then we heal.

What I watched was improvisation of an eighty-nine-year-old brain's organic accumulation of abnormally folded protein, translucence at the vortex of amyloid plaques and tangles. But it was also a repertory, a ball masque, a mixer, which in Mimi's case was a cotillion ball during debutante season. It was an affair we all lovingly showed up for, perfectly unprepared and all wearing the wrong shoes.

It was *Our Dance With Dementia* that lasted five-and-a-half terribly beautiful years.

CPSIA information can be obtained
at www.ICGtesting.com
Printed in the USA
BVHW03s0828220818
525294BV00001B/30/P